# SIMP...

# SIMPLY REAL

Your Guide to Creating a Happier
Life in an Easy and Relaxed Way

Karla J. Henry

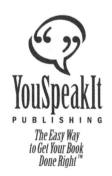

YouSpeakIt
PUBLISHING
The Easy Way
to Get Your Book
Done Right™

ISBN: 978-1-945446-90-0

*This book is dedicated to the hope
that we may all find that life can be lived
from an easy and relaxed space.*

.

# Contents

# Acknowledgments

I am grateful and appreciate the Holy Spirit within, always there, ever present, loving, supporting, and guiding me.

I am grateful and appreciate my entire life's journey. I am able to say this now, based on what I know today.

I am grateful for my family: Mom, Dad, and Nicki. My relationship with them led me into *me* and the power and possibilities within.

I am grateful and appreciate the teachings of Abraham Hicks, who first introduced me to the Law of Attraction, helping me to understand how to live and experience a more fun and fulfilled life.

I am grateful for my teachers on this life journey: my mentor, Pat Ramsay; my coaches: Gina Devee, Joshua Rosenthal and the Integrative Nutrition family, Tasha Chen, Gladys Diaz, and Michelle Roza; and my sister-friends: Dainia Baugh, Franciene Chin, Gillian Ferguson, and Jackie Domenico.

I am grateful to all my clients for allowing me to support their desire to change, evolve, and expand their lives.

I am grateful to YouSpeakIt Publishing for providing me the opportunity to complete my book in an easy and relaxed way.

# Introduction

I am Karla, a spirit being residing in a body that is currently living on the beautiful island of Jamaica. I have learned to be open and at ease with myself. I have learned to create my life, moment by moment, and to have fun while doing it. In this book, I will share with you how you can create your life in this same way.

Do you find yourself unable to forgive people for pain you've experienced in the past?

Is *un*forgiveness keeping you from living a happy life?

I have been able to forgive and bring acceptance to my own childhood traumas as an adult, and as a result, I have found a way to more deeply claim and acknowledge the power within me. You can find this power as well.

I live a life of ease and fun now, but it wasn't always this way. I was once terribly frustrated with the hardships in my life, which to me at the time felt like failure. I felt I had gotten the short end of the stick in life. My glass felt empty. Something was definitely wrong with me. Those were my beliefs.

I was failing at life and I couldn't understand why.

I started researching self-help books, and in my reading, I stumbled upon a coach by the name of Gina DeVee. I listened to her and her message resonated with me. I knew I wanted to work with her. Somehow, I figured out how I was going to afford her twelve-month program, Divine Living Academy, and I signed up.

During that group program, Gina touched on some topics that pushed some of my buttons, and it hurt. I was ashamed to share my feelings in front of the group. I remembered and relived quite a bit of pain from my childhood—not feeling loved, feeling unworthy, feeling alone. I spoke to a close friend of mine about these feelings, and he recommended that I do therapy with a psychologist. And because the person I am is always wanting to improve, I did not hesitate.

The therapeutic modalities that the psychologist chose for me became a catalyst for change. In short, we didn't talk my issues to death. It ended up being exactly what I needed to accept, forgive, and transform.

I wanted to transform, full stop. So, I went from coaching to therapy; then I narrowed my scope and got my holistic coaching certification from the Institute of Integrative Nutrition. I was attracted to the teachings of Abraham Hicks. These teachings lit—and continue to light—so many light bulbs in me. The more I studied, the more I understood. I became a believer in the Law of Attraction.

To go even deeper, I invested in a money coach, Tasha Chen, and the Science of Getting Rich Academy. Oh, my dears, you need to know your mindset around money and abundance must be healed in order for money and abundance to flow in an easy, relaxed, and healthy way. If not, that is where the concept of *hard work equals success* comes from.

What I know for sure is that whenever I lean on the Spirit within me, wisdom, clarity, and help come to me on my journey. Learning to lean on the Spirit within has made my life easier, more relaxed, and more rewarding. So that is what I do.

I wanted to attract the right man for me, so I examined my past relationships in light of my new knowledge. I realized I wasn't attracting the right and best man for me, so I invested in relationship coaches. As I am writing this book, I am currently working with The Love Twins: Gladys and Michelle, in their program, Ready to Love Again. I know I am truly a work in progress, and this will never stop because I am always growing and evolving into the woman I deserve to be.

I wrote this book because I wanted to share my journey with you. I wanted to give voice to *me* and be made visible and to help you in the process. I have so much to share about my own ah-ha moments and my transformation. Writing this book is a good way to reach more people.

My hope is that this book will support you and help you fill in the gaps in your life, or maybe just make your light shine brighter. Life doesn't have to be so hard and complicated. It is our beliefs and thoughts that add the hard energy to our lives. You can create the life of your dreams in an energy of ease and fun.

Start believing.

# CHAPTER ONE

---

# Loving Yourself
# Despite Your Childhood

## FORGIVENESS—LETTING GO

Forgiveness is the first step on the path to healing, to moving forward, and beginning to manifest whatever desires you have. However, forgiveness is only for you.

I will repeat that. *Forgiveness is only for you.* It is never about the person you are forgiving. Forgiveness is not for the other person; forgiveness is for *you.*

We cannot hold on to the energy of *un*forgiveness. It is like luggage, a heavy piece of baggage packed with all our hurts. It weighs us down, and after a while, it creates other dis-eases in our bodies and in our lives. As I have said before and will say again, forgiveness is not for the other person; forgiveness is for you.

I am going to tell you a story in this book. As I tell it, I will be remembering this story in terms of forgiveness.

For a long time, I blamed my parents for their mistakes, and I blamed them for my failures. I blamed them for where I was. I did not allow the peace of forgiveness to heal me. I needed to learn that forgiveness is not for them, as I have said. It is for me.

The truth is that my parents operated from what they knew at the time and from their own life experiences. Yes, we always have the choice to do better. But sometimes, we just don't. When we act from what we know at the time, we may repeat a negative cycle. This is the way a *generational curse* may continue to impact families. To break the curse, someone needs to break the pattern.

When I was graduating from high school in Jamaica, there was a school policy put in place that made passing religious studies one of the requirements to get a diploma. I attended a Catholic high school, the same school my mother had gone to as well. I did not pass that class. I find that so ironic now that I am so spiritual and connected to knowing I have this huge amazing energy inside of me we call God, the Universe, Source, or the Divine. However, back then, I didn't pass the class, so I wasn't eligible for a diploma, only for what they called a school-leaving certificate.

It was devastating to me. I felt completely unsupported by my parents, who didn't fight for me, although my mother had a relationship with the school. I wasn't a poor student academically. It was just religion that was my downfall—so I wasn't happy with God either.

When I went to graduation, in front of the entire school, in front of all the parents, I didn't get a diploma. I felt so embarrassed, so ashamed, so hurt, and so alone. I probably would have felt less embarrassed if the school-leaving certificate was placed in the same black holder as the diploma. No one would have noticed. However, it was a rolled-up piece of paper with a blue ribbon that was handed to me, and it was obvious to everyone there I had failed to achieve a diploma.

In the current generation, it's not uncommon for parents to show up for their children and fight for them, but I don't think my parents and their generation experienced that kind of support, and that's part of the reason they didn't support me. But be that as it may, that feeling of being unloved and unsupported was something I took along with me for a very long time. In retrospect, I think that lack of support was the reason I had difficulties with my relationships, whether personal or work. I had such a problem connecting to anything that meant something to me because of my fear of being hurt and rejected.

I had trouble letting go of those feelings and forgiving them. I also did not allow myself to understand that they knew only what they knew at that time. Most importantly, I never even expressed to them that I was carrying this hurt. I could not even acknowledge the hurt out loud.

In retrospect, I see that, as a result, I punished myself for way too long and the release of this punishment didn't come until many years later. It took some time, understanding, and compassion, but eventually, I was able acknowledge my feelings and find forgiveness.

## Breaking the Cycle of Pain

It was over twenty years later when I started to ask myself the questions I needed to ask to begin the process of healing:

*Why did I keep repeating certain cycles in my life?*

*Why is it I quit things so quickly?*

*Why was it so hard for me to find and keep good relationships?*

The cycle of hurt had to be broken in order for me to heal and move forward. The generational curse had to stop with me. I had to acknowledge the hurt and let it go, and this could only start with forgiveness — forgiveness of *me* first, for all the crap I did to others and to myself, and then forgiveness of my parents. They did the best they knew at the time.

I learned a great deal about forgiveness by working with my relationship coaches, Gladys and Michele. I am very happy and grateful to have found this new kind of wisdom and clarity, and now, I am truly appreciative of my parents. It's because of this transformation that I am able to be their caregiver today. Though little reminders of the hurt will sometime pop up, they do not stay long because I know how to revert to forgiveness and the letting go. God is good to me.

---

### Talking Yourself Through Forgiveness

I learned this practice from my relationship coaches, Gladys and Michelle. You can use it for any kind of forgiveness. In this example, I share my responses for dealing with the feeling of being unloved.

Ask yourself these questions:

- *Am I unloved forever? Am I not going to be chosen forever?* – NO!

- *If I let this go today what becomes possible for me?* – I can feel happier: fun, laughter. I can feel more relaxed: at ease and be in gratitude.

---

- *Am I ready to move past this fear?* YES. Now when the fear pops up, and it will, tell yourself: *It's not true. I will be chosen. I will be loved.* Speak to the fear. Do not accept what you don't deserve. It will be so much better.

- *If this fear were to actually happen (never being chosen), what is the worst thing that could happen?* — BEING ALONE!

- *What scares me about being alone?* Maybe: UNLOVED, UNSUPPORTED

- *What scares me about being unloved?* I DON'T MATTER.

- *Is what I am afraid of happening now?* NO. Our fears are future-based, and we get to shift those thoughts to a better feeling in the now.

### Perspective: Seeing the Hand That Was Dealt

I mentioned before that my parents were working only with the hand they had been dealt. Without any judgment, that is the perspective I found for myself. This perspective enabled me to see the situation more clearly and realize I couldn't keep punishing them. I couldn't keep having bad thoughts about them. My truth is that when I was living my life that way, I was punishing myself with their mistakes. I was only creating more pain.

I had to get a new picture, a new perspective of them and me. I had to decide I wanted to be better and do better. It was a decision I made. At that time, my parents only knew how to love based on how they were loved. That is what we show our children.

Yes, thank God for technology and social media and the internet and all the information available to us today, but back then, we did not have all that information. In addition, back then, we didn't share our journeys with each other to help each other know what it was that we needed to do.

So, we all need to look at what the other person's hand looks like. I am not making excuses for them, but what I am saying is you have the ability to understand and apply some compassion. Then, you can form a different perspective. You can say to yourself: *Okay, that is what they knew how to do. I know better, so I can do better.*

It is a transformational process. It will not happen overnight; at least that was not my experience. It took time, commitment, and resounding patience with myself.

## It's a Daily Practice

The daily practice is literally a practice of awareness. It is about being present with how you are feeling at any given moment. I use it for whatever is coming up for me at the time. A daily practice is something said or done in order to let some feelings go so we don't carry them into the following day.

When I go to bed at night, before I go to sleep, I often find there are issues on my mind that I need to put a light on. I simply focus on the issue and ask: *Okay, how can I view this a different way?*

In most cases, it is not about me, but it is to acknowledge how I am feeling about something. That is the most important aspect of the daily practice. It is to acknowledge how you are feeling in that moment and to release the pieces that are not serving you or aren't meant for you.

## My Daily Practice of Forgiving and Letting Go

Before I close my eyes at night, I go over my day and look for aspects of the day that were not that great. I quietly review what happened and forgive the situation, the person, and myself. Then I visualize a reset button and press it to set an intention for a better day tomorrow.

For me, it is also important to ask God to relieve me of the burden of *un*forgiveness. I must also state that, at times, something may happen that triggers a not-so-good feeling and response and, in the moment, once I am aware, I will go into forgiveness. I was not always able to do this. It can really only happen when awareness has been practiced so much that it's now just what you do.

## I AM ENOUGH

You have probably heard somewhere about the importance of knowing that you are enough and that you are worthy. These words are simple, but they have profound importance.

Do you believe that you are enough?

Do you think you are worthy of having a good life? Of being happy?

You must know in your heart that you matter. If you don't know you matter, then you will take anything that comes your way in life, even the not so good things, the negatives, the pain, and the hurt. If you don't believe you are deserving of something better, then you will not experience God's best for you.

*I praise you, for I am fearfully and wonderfully made.*
*Wonderful are your works; my soul knows it very well.*
— Psalm 139:14 (NAB)

Therefore, you are perfectly and wonderfully made and you are enough.

## Finding Faith and Self-Worth

As I've told you, at my high school graduation, instead of getting a high school diploma, I received a school-leaving certificate. Apart from the embarrassment I felt, I also thought, at the time, that my life wasn't going to amount to much because I didn't have a diploma. For me, a high school diploma was the beginning of what would be possible in life. Without it, I didn't know what to do next.

When I had the opportunity to leave Jamaica in 1988, I saw it as a chance to start anew, and I took it. Not only was I leaving Jamaica the island, I was also leaving my parents, my sister, my friends, and everything I knew. But that didn't perturb me one bit. I felt at that time there had to be more for me and going to the United States was a great opportunity. It was the land where dreams come true — or so I'd heard. It turned out to be the right decision.

Long story short: My aunt, the one I lived with, encouraged me to go to Rutgers University admissions office on the New Brunswick campus and apply as a walk-in. And that I did. I walked in with my school-leaving certificate and my high school transcripts and the examination certificates I had received in Jamaica. That was all I had. I did not even have SAT scores.

As I sat down in front of the dean, I remember feeling a growing sense of hope. I could see new possibilities for my future. Little did I know that was all I needed — that little bit of faith in myself. A small part of me knew I wanted to be great and do great things. That small part was strong and certain, although the bigger part of me was still struggling with not feeling I mattered or was worthy of this greatness.

The lack of support from my parents still weighed heavily upon me, but as I sat in front of the dean, and he accepted my application into the university, everything began to change. That is when I started to feel like there was something special about me and I actually mattered.

Most of us, if not all, are shaped by the opinions of our parents. What our parents think of us matters. Theirs are the opinions we grow up caring about the most, so what they think can set up a belief system that persists within us. If we are not careful, we may end up believing what others say about us is the truth.

It can actually be the truth if it aligns with who you believe you are, positive or negative. When you don't have love and support, the feeling that says *I matter* or *I am worthy* is not there, and we kind of feel doomed.

But in that moment with the dean, I began to regain the hope that I actually mattered. I felt I was worthy of what was going to happen to me next.

## Self-Talk: Paying Attention to Your Voices

When you are lacking love and support, this lack can plant seeds of insecurity inside you. What you hear from the people around you, including your parents, may become your internal voice as well.

What do the voices inside say to you?

Because I heard a lot of criticism, my voices were extremely critical. Those seeds took root in my mind until my internal voices were full of criticism. *I was too fat. I would never be a leader. I would always be a follower. My voice doesn't matter.* I heard those voices because those I most cared about had told me these things. I needed to reprogram myself so I could change what those voices were saying.

To me, those internal voices are really the ego, and most times, the ego is not at all speaking for our edification. Often, what it says to me is negative and defeating. I realized I needed to find a better perspective. I began to practice being aware of what I was hearing and what I was telling myself. I had to learn to be present with my thoughts. Once I became aware, I came to the understanding that I could start to change my perspective at that moment. I could change those voices.

Once I heard something, I could say to myself: *Oh, no that is not it, that is not who I am.* Then, I could change what the voice was saying: *That's not who I am. I am this . . .*

Make sure you acknowledge these thoughts because they will keep coming. They will always come; they are like weeds. However, if we acknowledge the negative and defeating thoughts, we can literally pluck each of them out and replace them with something more positive and in alignment with who we believe we are.

Learning to be present with your thoughts will be discussed further in Chapter Two. Stay tuned.

## Affirmations

Affirmations are positive *now* statements about life — statements in the present tense. They can reflect who you are now or who you desire to be.

Affirmations can and should be used anytime, especially if thoughts of doubt or fear are apparent. An affirmation helps to reinforce in a positive way what you want to see happen and or feel in any given moment.

Affirmations are more effective when I say them out loud versus in my head. When spoken, I allow myself to hear and feel the energy of what I am believing. If I do not believe what I am affirming, I will make the statement into one that is more believable. For instance, if I look in the mirror and I don't like what I see, saying "I am beautiful" maybe hard for me to believe in that moment. So, I find a better-feeling thought and say something like, "I am an awesome person," or "I am enough."

I suggest writing out your affirmations and keeping them handy so they become easily accessible in a time of need. For instance, stick them on your bathroom mirror or refrigerator or keep them in your car. After doing this for a while, you will notice you just know what affirmations to reach for that will make you feel instantly better.

Of all the affirmations I have learned and read about, the ones that really resonate with me and have helped me are the ones I've done from a place of faith.

You might have heard the saying: *Fake it 'til you make it.*

I prefer to say instead: *FAITH it 'til you make it.*

When I am using affirmations, I speak to myself as if whatever I wish has already happened. I look at my life to find what I wish for, and I express gratitude. For

instance, if I don't feel beautiful, I look fo
about me. I might say to myself: *I am gr.
hands. They help me write my dreams. I am gr.
beautiful heart that supports my body.*

I always start with *I am.* I start with *I am* because I
believe in the power of what those two words can do;
they create. *I am* lights the way to where you desire to
go. So, it is whatever you want it to be.

My affirmations are always positive. I don't ever use
an *I am* statement with negativity because that is not
what I am looking for in my life. For example, I am not
going to say *I am broke* when I really want to say I have
more than enough. We can always find abundance in
other things than money.

**Here are some examples of positive affirmations:**

- *I am happy and grateful now, in an easy and relaxed manner, in a healthy and positive way.*

- *I am enough.*

- *I am doing the best I can.*

- *I am getting stronger and healthier at my ideal weight.*

- *I am amazing.*

- *I am a good friend.*

- *I am loving and lovable.*

- *I am wisdom, and I always know what to do next.*

- *I am at the right place, at the right time, doing the right thing.*

- *I am a good listener.*

- *I am reliable.*

- *I am a good steward over my money.*

- *I am in perfect health.*

- *I am flexible in my body.*

- *I am feeling free in time, money, health, and relationships.*

- *I am feeling grateful and appreciative of all things.*

- *I am feeling courageous and bold.*

- *I am excited about this day.*

- *I am worthy of the things I desire.*

- *I am feeling happy to just BE today.*

- *I am feeling loved by God/The Divine.*

- *I am love.*

- *I am happy with me.*

- *I am feeling excited to serve my ideal and right clien.. today.*

- *I am feeling capable and equipped to do this.*

## TIME IS STILL ON YOUR SIDE

Life puts so much pressure on us to get this and that done by such and such time. We tell ourselves things like: *It's too late; I'm too old; It's not going to happen.*

I have fallen prey to that on many occasions, but I have come to believe that God, the Universe, Source, the Divine can actually speed up time; can make things happen in a day. It is incumbent upon us to ask, believe, and prepare to receive what we desire. It is in the believing without wavering that you are made ready for the thing you desire. It is the believing that determines how fast time moves.

My belief here is that the answer to my *ask* can be *yes* or *not now,* but it can also be *something better,* and this just elevates my faith even further.

An example that I like to use and share with my friends is about our culture's attitude toward retirement. Our society has taught that you should be saving for retirement from the time you start your first job. For those of us who have none, it kind of feels doomy,

dark. It feels like when you retire you
ything.

tead, is aligned with Jeremiah 29:11 (NIV):

*"For ı know the plans I have for you," declares
the Lord, "Plans to prosper you and not to harm
you, plans to give you hope and a future."*

Do what you actually love; serve and have a really
great time doing it. Time is of no value to God because
God's plans and timing are not humans'. For instance,
what may take five years to accomplish in humans'
own strength, with God's guidance may just take one
year.

In Psalm 90:4 (NIV), Moses used a simple yet profound
analogy in describing the timelessness of God:

*For a thousand years in Your sight
are like a day that has just gone by,
or like a watch in the night.*

God transcends time, and so we must not limit an
infinite God to our time schedule. Therefore, if you
believe this like I do, then time is still on your side.

It's never too late to start over!

## Who Says It's Too Late?

Age is but a number. Everything comes back to how you feel. That is where your energy is, and that is how you create your life.

It's all about your emotions and the way you feel about yourself; if you are feeling old, then don't be surprised if that's the life you start to experience. Old. But if you are feeling young, bright, and hopeful, then you are going to keep living an amazing life. That is how I feel right now.

The pressure we put on ourselves to get everything done by a certain time is not necessary. Think about the pressure women put on themselves when it comes to having children. Yes, I understand our bodies, and that we really don't want to be having children after a certain age because of the energy it requires.

However, this idea that your biological clock is ticking can be such pressure. If you believe in putting yourself under that pressure, then so be it. I have never believed it, and I have friends who have never believed it, friends who are older and still having children safely. So, it really comes back to your belief, the energy behind your belief, and how much you are standing firm with that belief. Jay Shetty often quotes the proverb below:

> *Every delay has its blessings.*
> ~ Arabic Proverb

Who says it's too late? Not the Universe!

## The Universe Has Your Back

Everyone's path is going to be different. If you continue to live your life by following other people and society, you are listening to *their* perspective, not *yours*. What other people think and believe is for them. It is not necessarily for you. You don't have to follow other people's beliefs.

What do you believe for *you?*

It all comes back to what you believe and what you desire. Whatever you believe is what you need to believe. Concentrate on all that you want, desire, and hope for. That thought-space is sacred. Your beliefs must be concrete and focused. Know that once you have that focus and you make your request known to God, to Source, then it has to happen.

At the start of 2017, I knew I was going to be turning fifty in October, and I wanted to go Europe. I also knew I wanted to travel in a first-class manner, and I wanted to have a certain amount of money with me. Wherever I stayed and however I traveled, I wanted to be comfortable, and I wanted to experience an easy, relaxed, and fun trip.

I checked out the cost of everything. I engaged a money coach, and she told me to start a *FUN* account, so that's exactly what I did; I was obedient, remembering that money must have a direction to flow to. I made sure the account was purposed entirely for fun. This bank account, as well as my research, was to show God I was serious about my desire to go Europe with all the bells and whistles I know I deserve.

You might be wondering if I was questioning how I was going to do it all. Actually, the *how* wasn't part of my thinking at all.

We need to be okay with leaving the *how* in the hands of the universe.

I understood that trying to figure out the *how* was not going to get me anywhere. Focusing on the *how*, I would have gotten bogged down in all the difficulties with questions like:

*How could I possibly achieve this objective?*

*How would I accumulate enough money in such a short amount of time?*

*How many pieces of business would have to be generated to get the amount of money that I wanted?*

I knew it would be too much, and I would have been stressed to no end. It would have been too daunting. So,

I journaled what I wanted. I journaled the experience as if I had already taken the trip. I journaled how the trip made me feel. In the FUN account, my coach told me to put any amount of money that felt good to me. It could sometimes be just loose change. Any extra money that came, I put in there.

Now the fun account did not generate the entire amount of money I needed; it wasn't supposed to. I showed faith by making deposits regularly and believing that the money would be multiplied. Every time thoughts of the *how* came to mind, I would speak to them quickly and affirm God had my back and would do exceedingly abundantly for me.

## God Is the Author of the *How*

Closer to my birthday, I went to the travel agency with some friends who planned on coming on a part of the trip with me. Because I live in a small country where everybody knows everybody, some other friends knew about my travel plans and the travel agency I planned to use. The travel agent, while discussing the best route to London and France said I could get an upgrade on the premium economy ticket I knew I had enough money for and had made peace with. I won't lie, though—I was still believing in first-class travel despite what my bank account said.

The agent was being quite guarded with her explanation of the upgrade, which I still thought was free until I asked, and she surprised me by saying "Karla, somebody gifted you an entire first-class trip to all the countries that you want to go to."

I was in shock. I went straight into gratitude; I even did a little praise dance in the office. Everybody in that travel agency stopped to hear my testimony on God having my back. For God is truly the author of the *how*.

That was my birthday gift, unbeknownst to me. I didn't know where it came from until later when the giver of the gift was revealed. With the business I had done during the year, I was able to earn all the cash I wanted to take with me on that trip. That is how I know the universe has my back.

When I had checked out the cost of everything initially, imagine if I had given up, thinking that *the how*, in my finite mind, seemed impossible. Instead, I was able to keep my fiftieth birthday trip dream alive, and it exceeded my expectations.

*Thank you, God.*

## You Are Doing the Best You Can

You don't have to be perfect.

This whole idea and concept of perfection is another pressuring piece for a lot of us, including me as I am writing this. It's the idea that whatever I'm doing needs to be perfect; I need to be perfect, whatever that may look like for me at the moment.

You may be looking at what you're doing right now, and it might not seem perfect. Give yourself the freedom to know you are doing the best you can right now.

Say it to yourself: *I am just doing the best I can right now.*

When you're working on a multi-step process, and you become fixated on the imperfections in one of your steps, this fixation can keep you from moving forward at all. If you are doing your best, acknowledge that. Focus on the good parts of your process, be grateful, and keep moving. Get it done. Done is better than perfect; it's a better-feeling place to be. And, after all, we can always revise and improve.

Always acknowledge when you are doing your best. It helps to alleviate the pressure of having to be perfect, and it can give you such ease when you are in the middle of a life struggle, things are falling apart, or you are under tremendous stress. If you allow, it will give you a healthier perspective just to say: *I am just doing the best I can do right now.*

# CHAPTER TWO

---

# Learning to Stand for Who You Are

## AWARENESS

Awareness is the state of being conscious of how you feel in the here and now. Whatever you are experiencing, you must pay attention to how you are feeling.

Are your thoughts causing you to feel good — or not good?

Acknowledge the feeling you have. If you have to change it, bless it, and then affirm a better-feeling thought. If you are enjoying the feeling in that moment, use that awareness to continue being that way.

### How Do You Feel Right Now?

That is a question most of us don't ask. We ask each other, "How are you?" Sometimes we wait for the answer and genuinely hear the response, but other times we aren't really listening. When asked, we often automatically say, "I am fine," but what does that really mean? We don't ever seem to cue in to how we are feeling.

We have to stop and ask ourselves, on a deeper level, how we are truly feeling in any given moment. That feeling identifies the emotional vibrational state that we are in at that moment. Asking the question is the key to being aware of how we are truly feeling.

Are you feeling well? Or not?

## Being Present With Your Thoughts and Feelings

Life is happening all the time, but it can happen *to us* or *for us*. We have to choose.

What have you chosen?

If you aren't sure, read the questions below:

- Do you just accept any old thing that comes along?

- Do you accept whatever state, negative or positive, that you find yourself in?

- Would you describe yourself as always responding by *rolling with the punches*, with no particular attention paid to your emotions or well-being?

If this sounds like you, it is likely that you are allowing life to simply happen to you. Instead, as I said, life can happen *for you*. The forward part of living this way requires some extra thinking, attention, and, most important, perspective.

When you are faced with a situation, instead of simply accepting it, you can ask yourself:

- *Is there a different way I can see this situation?*
- *Can I respond to the situation in a better way?*
- *What thoughts and actions would make me feel better?*

This is being present; this is awareness.

Often, you are going to have to talk to yourself to find new perspectives. You may find yourself talking to yourself out loud, and that's okay too. I talk to myself out loud all the time. I do it for emphasis when affirming so that the affirmation can take root in me.

I know they say crazy people talk to themselves. Well, am I crazy to want to feel well? No, and neither are you. If we don't speak into our own lives, who will?

## Ways to Become More Present

One of my favorite ways to become more present is to be *in gratitude*. Gratitude for *the now* and gratitude in appreciation of what is coming—as if I already have it—giving full attention to what is happening around me.

In a nutshell, treat your present as a new experience. Even if it feels like an old experience, your current perception of it can evoke a different feeling, which in turn will make you experience the moment differently.

For example, suppose I travel the same route each day as I drive to work. Every day, I encounter delays, traffic, horns honking, and it would be natural to experience some frustration.

But how can I experience this differently?

For me, I tend to start by observing my breath. In that moment, as I'm observing my breath, I usually start to become more aware of my surroundings. I am still in my car, and I am still in traffic, but now I notice there are trees along the road.

I am a fan of trees and I immediately begin to feel better. As I continue to breathe, I feel the movement of the trees and the leaves, and I begin to create this vision of them waving to me or smiling with me, and that helps to change the state that I am in. Instead of a state of frustration, I soon find myself in a state of gratitude.

If observing your breath isn't appealing to you, sing out loud. The simple act of singing can change your state and help you become more present with how you are feeling; it can bring you back to a happy state. From there, move yourself directly into gratitude.

You can go into a state of gratitude by being grateful for your surroundings, your job, your business, your family — all the things that make up that wonderful life you live.

## SELF-TALK

I grew up hearing that if I talk to myself or listen to myself talk in my head then I must be having some mental health issue. However, the older I've gotten, the more I've realized the importance of speaking to myself. We all have thoughts that are running all around in our minds, thoughts that are good, not good, or indifferent, and we need to address them. If not, they can — and will — take over your experience in a second. Remember, the most important relationship you will ever have is the one with *yourself*.

God responds to your belief. As I said earlier, what you believe, and what you are steadfast about, is what the Universe responds to.

## Spotting the Devil on Your Shoulder

Most of us have been socialized to believe that we toggle between two forces — an angel and a devil — one on each shoulder. I have come to understand that these forces are actually my own thoughts.

If I pay attention to the energy each thought projects, I can usually tell which one is for me. I can see which one is more aligned with who I really am: a spirit made in the image and likeness of God. That's the whole truth to me.

When I don't pay attention to my thoughts, I notice that, left unchecked, the other energy that we may call our ego — that negative voice — leads me into doubting who I am and the dreams I have for myself. This takes me down a path that is not fun, that is not easy or relaxed, a path where there is no grace at all. On this path, I am angered easily, and the day just spirals into one big mess.

Can you relate?

I recommend talking to yourself. It can help you to choose a better path, and it is great therapy; take it from me!

You believe what you say to yourself, so why not speak life and greatness into your life?

## Pay Attention to What's Being Said

Having conversations with yourself takes practice. I used to just react to whatever was coming my way without ever gaining an insight into whether it was for me or by me, and how my reaction could impact someone else.

Thoughts are streaming through our heads a mile a minute. These thoughts say a huge variety of things. Some are simple and some are complicated; some are gentle and some are hard; some are kind and some are unkind to me and to others. This is why paying attention is crucial to our well-being.

You are the creator of your reality, and your mind is the tool. Simply put, *thoughts become reality.*

This starts in your childhood. As Gordana Biernat wrote:

> You allowed [your deepest thoughts and beliefs about yourself], unconditionally, into your mind during your early childhood. You did this by mirroring your parents, siblings and neighbors — long before you could speak and "translate" your thoughts into conscious words and concepts.[1]

1 Biernat, Gordana. "Pay Attention to Your Thoughts." *Psychology Today.* March 2, 2018. psychologytoday.com/us/blog/the-essence-consciousness/201803/pay-attention-your-thoughts

Add these childhood influences to your experiences with school, work, social media, news, and so on, and you are basically living a life created by someone else. It is a life that has been manifested *through you* but not *by you.*

Biernat continues:

> Your beliefs "speak" directly to your subconscious mind which is entangled on a deep level of realty, with the very fabric of the Universe. Your thoughts are thus not insignificant. They are important because you are interacting with a conscious Universe which not only "hears" what you say but more importantly *knows* what you feel and *believe.* And the rule is—What you believe, you receive.[2]

This is exactly what I believe.

## Activating Your Voice to Stand for Who You Are

*Above all else, guard your heart,*
*for everything you do flows from it.*
~ Proverbs 4:23 (NIV)

Have you ever had a thought that just wasn't nice? A thought that was unkind? A thought that made you cringe with a feeling of guilt or remorse?

---

2 Biernat, 2018.

We all have thoughts like this from time to time. What matters is how we respond to the thought.

Do you discuss the thought? Do you pretend it did not happen?

These thoughts are like weeds, and if left unattended, they will take over and destroy the beautiful garden of our minds.

How can we stand up to these weed-thoughts?

- First, stop them in their tracks.

- Next, declare that there is no place for such thoughts in your mind.

- Finally, replace each of these thoughts with a new thought that is more supportive of who you are.

This may sound difficult, but you can do it. No matter what you are going through, you can focus on what is good.

Think about this: *What is going well for you in your life now?*

Even if it's only one thing, celebrate that one thing. The more you celebrate, the more you are in gratitude, and the more things will come into your life for you to celebrate and appreciate. There's always beauty around us in abundance. Seeing that abundance is what will activate your own feeling of abundance, despite what may be lacking in your life. It will shift your frequency to a higher level, which will allow you to see what's possible.

Again I say, try it. You won't be disappointed. Message me and tell me how this works for you. Look at the trees and what they offer you. Make a decision to smile at everyone you come into contact with. These are the many ways you can activate your voice to stand for who you are. That is straight power right there!

## COMMITMENT TO YOURSELF

There has been a lot of talk about self-love, loving ourselves, and putting ourselves first. There is so much truth and honor in doing that.

After all, if you are not committed to yourself, then who is?

Who is committed to your well-being? YOU.

Who is more committed to loving and caring for you than anybody else? YOU.

### Love of Self

Do I love me? Do you love you?

When was the last time you said *I love you* to yourself?

Love for self will determine how you talk to yourself and how you feed and move your body. Women may find it particularly difficult to be loving toward themselves. By nature, women tend to be very nurturing to others and giving of self, but many find it challenging to receive support and love from others, or even give themselves the gift of love. Some may interpret love of self as being selfish.

On the contrary, love of self demonstrates your well-being and happiness. If you love and value yourself, this means you will not settle for less than you deserve. You will have a positive view of yourself and will be confident of your place in this life. When you make mistakes, this confidence will help you not be too hard on yourself while you fix them. Courage and strength, which tend to be byproducts of operating in self-love, will help you face adversity.

## Engaging in Things That Make You Feel Good

What are you doing now?

Yes, I know you are reading this book — but seriously — are you engaging in stuff that makes you feel good?

It is so easy to get bogged down in the day-to-day humdrum of life, and that state can lead us into accepting and doing things that just don't light us up.

Can you find something to do that makes you smile? I know you can.

## Put Your Mask on First

When flight attendants give safety instructions before take-off, you hear them say that, if oxygen masks drop down, you must put your mask on first before you assist anyone else. There is a reason for this and it can be lifesaving. It makes sense that if you can't breathe, you can't help anyone else. You have to get yourself some oxygen before you give of yourself to others.

Let's think of this as a metaphor. The oxygen can take the form of whatever you need to be happy and healthy. You must fill your cup first, before you can help others.

What would you like to fill your cup with? Love, time, positive energy, happiness?

Fill your cup. Then, and only then, can you truly show up with a strength that will support others.

# CHAPTER THREE

---

# Visualization and *Feelization*

## DEFINITIONS OF VISUALIZATION AND *FEELIZATION*

I have read many definitions of visualization and *feelization*. You may also have read about these concepts before. Let me give you my perspective.

### Visualization

Of the many definitions of visualization I have read, I like this one most:

> *Visualization is simply a mental rehearsal.*
> *You create mental images in your mind*
> *of having or doing whatever it is that you want.*[3]
> ~ John Kehoe

In my estimation, visualization is a form of dreaming. Sometimes it takes the form of closing your eyes and seeing a picture of what you desire. However, you can

---

3 learnmindpower.com/using-mind-power/visualizations/

also visualize with your eyes open. It is about getting in touch with how you *want* to picture something. When visualizing something, I focus on the way I want to experience it in my imagination. I can even go as far as engaging all my senses — sight, smell, hearing, taste, and touch — in the visualization.

It is like ordering a meal that you have been dreaming about; if you allow yourself to go deeply into that experience, you can almost taste and smell it. Plus, you will feel your body get ready to enjoy it. You just know it is going to be good.

Visualizing is a good way to help organize thoughts and reduce stress, but it is also a way of attracting what you want. What you focus on, you attract.

Remember, *faith it until you make it*. Pretend you have what you desire. Your subconscious mind doesn't know the difference. Focus on what you want in such detail that the Universe has to conspire to bring it you. Pay attention and listen for cues so you know the next step to take.

### *Feel*ization: A New Concept

Feelization has been defined as "the mental creation of feelings of physical emotion or of feeling oneself execute a skill or a program in the mind by the power of thought and imagination."[4]

In the last section, we talked about how to ˅  ̣ ̣ ̣d enjoy the process of visualization. Feelization allows you to take it a step further. You will add emotions, feelings, and good vibes to the visualization exercise.

To begin, ask yourself: *How is the visual making you feel?*

Go deeper than just answering *good*. It is in deepening your focus on your energy around having this desire that it will become a reality.

Suppose you want a healthier body. Instead of focusing on the health issue, you could focus on being healthy.

First, visualize. What does that picture look like?

Once you have that healthy image of yourself, tune in to the feeling you get when that visual, that image has been formed. For example, you may feel *strong,* or *vibrant.* You may feel, *alive, thriving, young,* or *free.* Get the picture? That is feelization.

The vibrating energy and the creative forces coming from this exercise will then start to express your desire in your life. Once we understand this, we can begin to design — to create — our lives with loads of clarity and purpose in an easy and relaxed manner.

---

4 definition-of.com

## Now What?

1. Take the time to think on what you desire.

2. Write your desires down. I cannot stress enough the beauty and power of writing down your dreams.

3. Then, for each dream, each desire, write down how you think you will feel when you have what you desire. Make sure the feelings you want to experience are strong and positive and empowering. Be specific; don't just say *I want to feel good.*

See the list of feeling words from Jack Canfield in the feelings chart below (fig. 1) for some ideas. Have fun with it. Pay attention to the lightness and the smiles that come up when you think and feel.

| | | | | |
|---|---|---|---|---|
| Adored | Dynamic | Graceful | Noble | Spectacular |
| Alive | Eager | Gracious | Open | Strong |
| Amazing | Easy | Grateful | Optimistic | Tender |
| Appreciated | Empowered | Happy | Opulent | Terrific |
| Appreciative | Energized | Harmonious | Passionate | Thrilled |
| Awesome | Enlightened | Hopeful | Peaceful | Tranquil |

| | | | | |
|---|---|---|---|---|
| Blissful | Enthusiastic | Inspired | Playful | Trusting |
| Bold | Excited | Invigorated | Positive | Unlimited |
| Bright | Exhilarated | Irresistible | Powerful | Uplifted |
| Brilliant | Expanded | Jazzed | Precious | Valuable |
| Calm | Exquisite | Joyful | Proud | Vibrant |
| Cheerful | Extraordinary | Joyous | Quiet | Vivacious |
| Cherished | Exuberant | Jubilant | Radiant | Warm |
| Clear | Fabulous | Juicy | Ready | Welcomed |
| Comfortable | Flowing | Kind | Receptive | Whole |
| Confident | Focused | Light | Refreshed | Wise |
| Content | Free | Lovable | Relaxed | Wonderful |
| Courageous | Frisky | Loving | Relieved | Worthy |
| Creative | Fun | Luxurious | Renewed | Yummy |
| Decisive | Glorious | Magical | Resilient | Zestful |
| Delicious | Glorious | Marvelous | Sensational | |
| Divine | Glowing | Miraculous | Serene | |

*Figure 1 Feelings Chart*[5]

5 jackcanfield.com/blog/affirmations/amp/

This is by no means a complete list, but it should give you some ideas. Remember; think about how you *want* to feel. This will determine your energy around your visual.

## THE VALUE OF COMBINING VISUALIZATION AND *FEEL*IZATION

Visualization makes it easy for you to see what you want, like, and desire. Feelization enables you to attach feelings of positive energy behind what you visualize. When you connect visualization and feelization, you have the added bonus of creating by feeling your way to what you desire. Feelization also enables you to assess whether your feelings match with your visualization.

Let's say I want a particular house. It's a popular style of house in a popular area. When I visualize myself with that house and everything else that goes with it, I realize that this house, though beautiful and in a good area, doesn't match the feelings I have when I think more deeply. The truth for me is that the visual of the house is not aligning with the feeling I want to experience. Maybe the upkeep of the house makes me feel less abundant. Maybe the commute to work is overwhelming. Maybe living in a big house complicates life instead of creating an experience of ease. Whatever the reason, it is clear to me that the feeling I have about the house does not match up with the visualization of my desire.

You must make a connection between what you want and how you feel, and that feeling must be believed. If you are not connected to how you feel about what you want, manifesting what you desire will be very difficult.

## Connection

Visualization activates the creative juices of the subconscious mind. From that practice, creative — even inspired — ideas will start to reveal themselves to you. From those ideas will come the inspired action (the next step) to be taken towards achieving your desires, intentions, and dreams. Inspired ACTION is where the power is versus you trying to figure out the how.

As author Jack Canfield wrote, the practice of visualization "activates the law of attraction, thereby drawing into your life the people, resources, and circumstances you will need to achieve your goals."[6]

When you're visualizing, you are effectively asking the Universe: *What do I do next?*

---

6 Canfield, Jack. "Visualization techniques to affirm your desired outcomes." jackcanfield.com/blog/visualize-and-affirm-your-desired-outcomes-a-step-by-step-guide

When you get an answer, pay attention, no matter how simple the answer is, and step into action.

## The Power Behind the Connection

The power behind these connections is our invisible resource, the inner guide that is available to every one of us. We may refer to that power by different names, like *the Universe, Source, the Divine,* or *God.*

As long as I put the time into visualizing and feeling my goals, my desires, and my intentions, and I surround myself with positive people and things that flood my mind with the glorious feelings I want to experience, this power will co-create with me. God will give me guidance. The Universe will make the next steps clear to me.

I love asking God for guidance. When I commit to my daily practice of visualizing and feeling, I feel inspired to move and to act in a direction toward what I want. It becomes an abundant and exciting experience. Try it. Tap into the super-conscious mind, the God-mind that's within each of us, the realm of perfect ideas.

What idea is just right for you in this moment?

Are you ready to ask the Universe? Are you ready to move?

The power behind the connection will not get expressed in our favor until we move. Take action, for we know that "faith without works is dead." (KJV, 2:14)

I prefer to move through inspiration. By that, I mean I ask God to reveal to me my next action step. I also will continue to take action steps, doing all that I can do, and be careful not to bring harm to others. That is my process.

## The Power of the Connection

I believe that everything I experience comes from within me. Everything comes from thoughts I have had — good and not so good — coupled with my energies that have manifested into reality. The key is to understand and know that you have the power of choice in every moment.

How do you want to feel right now?

Whatever you decide is your power of choice. It is simple. You can choose to feel good, to have a different perspective, a different visual that will evoke a more positive feeling or an improved feeling. It is all about doing your best in that moment with the superpower that is within you, the superpower that we all have at our disposal to help and guide us.

Along the way, be as gentle and loving with yourself as you can. I have had to be so present with this in my life. Gently remind yourself that you know, wholeheartedly, that you are doing the best you can. Remind yourself that you are taking a step in the best direction for you.

## HOW TO CONNECT FEELINGS TO THE VISUALS

As mentioned before, connecting feelings to the visual is all about adding energy, some good vibes, to what you are visualizing. In this section, we are going to be exploring how to create your own daily practice that will enable you to apply this process in your life.

### Establish a Daily Practice

You can practice connecting visualization and feelization in many ways. You must figure out what works for you. Whatever method you use, make it a daily practice.

To begin your daily practice, try following these basic steps:

1. Set your intentions.
2. Establish a regular practice time.
3. Establish a quiet place to work.
4. Check in to monitor how you are feeling.
5. Regularly look for evidence to support your intentions.

We'll talk more about each step below.

## Step 1: Set Your Intentions

In setting an intention, this is where you will get clear on what you want and why you want it. The *why* will anchor your commitment to sustaining the daily practice. For example, let's assume my intention is to commit to meditating for fifteen minutes every morning before I get out of bed. Now that I've set my intention, I need to find my *why*.

I ask myself: *What are the feelings I want to experience?*

If you need help on this step, you can review the feelings chart from Jack Canfield (see Figure 1, earlier in this chapter).

Here is my *why*: I want to commit to meditating because it makes me feel calm, have more clarity, and feel more appreciation for the day ahead. Those are the feelings I want to experience.

## Step 2: Establish a Regular Practice Time

In order to get the most out of this process, establish a daily practice time that you can maintain. In the morning, I intend for the day and at night, I go into gratitude and appreciation. Set a schedule in your calendar; that is *your* time.

In creating new habits, start out small. Be gentle and loving with yourself. As you begin to develop a rhythm and the enjoyment of this time, increase the time spent. Some days, it may take ten minutes and other days, thirty minutes or more. Have fun with it in an easy and relaxed manner.

## Step 3: Establish a Quiet Place to Work

If meditating is a daily practice, have a quiet space. Create a little spot that is just for you if you live with others. You can set up music and candles ahead of time. If you are into journaling, which I am — more on that later, have a notebook or journal and a pen on hand.

It can be beneficial to share your process and intentions with another person, but be sure it is a person who will support you. That person should be added to the energy to make the intention stronger, not weaker.

## Step 4: Check In to Monitor How You Are Feeling

You should be feeling those feelings you had intended in the beginning. If you are not enjoying the practice, make adjustments. Remember, it is your time and your practice; there is no right or wrong way, so do not judge yourself. There isn't a one-size-fits-all approach. Allow the Universe to give you ideas.

## Step 5: Look for Evidence
## That Supports Your Intentions

Throughout your day, look for evidence around you that supports your intentions and the feelings you wanted to experience. If you look from a place of being present in the moment, you will see and experience what you truly desire. Enjoy to the fullest.

## My Daily Practice

My daily practice includes two activities: meditating and journaling. I really love to journal. I use this practice as a tool to create my life.

In Habakkuk 2:2 (ESV), God said, "Write the vision; make it plain on tablets, so he may run who reads it."

I have interpreted the verse to mean that when I journal, God will move to co-create with me. Hence, what I write becomes real; I actually get to feel the dream. I feel my way to what I want through journaling. This process is so much fun, and my level of excitement and energy is usually quite high when I'm writing. I strongly recommend this kind of journaling.

I tend to start my journaling in a general space and then I get going with more details. I might write five, six, or seven pages of details and feelings. I always try to write as if I have already received what I want.

For example, here is part of a journal entry for the trip I took to Europe when I was turning fifty. My intention was to become or embody all that I was asking for regarding this birthday trip.

*It is September 20, 2017; I'm off to London and then Paris, and then wherever I feel led to go. I am so happy and grateful now for this trip and the abundance of good feelings I have. I love my business-class experience. I am comfortable, sated, and rested for when I land in London. I love the ease of going through the airport en route to Paris. All is well. I am so blessed and favored on this entire trip. All my flights are on time and everywhere I go people are wonderful and happy to see me — I feel so loved and welcomed to this side of the world.*

*I love that I'm with the girls, and I am feeling so deserving and abundant and rich. This trip makes me feel rich. My energy is feeling high the entire trip, and I am having the time of my life. The hotel in Paris is a good choice. My room is so special — clean, beautiful, and just right for me. I feel so comfortable and cozy.*

*I love the staff at the hotel. I feel so special. The staff at the airports and everywhere I go have been so friendly and nice. I feel worthy and seen. I am having fun and feel so good. I love the ease of the time in Paris. I love the ease of dining and shopping and traveling throughout this country. I am feeling my best. The Universe has really supported me on this trip and helped me create.*

*I love creating this abundant, rich-feeling experience. God is all good to me. So, Paris, thanks for the love. London, I get to meet you again. My time in London is an adventure. I am appreciating all the sights, the cafes, the food, the wine, the people. Life feels so good. My fiftieth feels fantastic. I feel the love of life and all those who have turned up for me.*

*This trip to eat, pray, and love has blessed me so much. This trip keeps giving to me and I'm grateful. I am so open to receiving all of what the Universe has for me. I am so happy and feel happy to be here. The environment is on my side. The trees and flowers are so beautiful. The weather feels amazing and supports me.*

*The cells of my body are thriving and supporting my body. I appreciate my body for supporting me and loving me on this trip. Thank you, my body. All is well. Things are always working out for me. Things have worked out for me on this trip. I am feeling so very abundant. My cup is overflowing and I have so much to give and am so open to receive all of God's goodness.*

*Everything I desire from this trip is so much more than I could have imagined or expected. Tours, events, experiences, new people, and sales — all manifest for* me. The Universe has my back for real and is shining brightly for me. Unexpected money, unexpected deals, unexpected surprises manifest for me. What a feeling of joy and satisfaction. I am playing and feeling expansive – so I should – because the Universe is abundant. Thank you, thank you, thank you God. I have manifested business class. I have manifested US$10k for this trip. I have manifested love. I have manifested new friends. I have manifested me in all my glory. I am feeling great, amazing, wonderful, and beautiful and abundant. Thank you, God. And so it is.

## Aligning Your Visuals With Your Feelings

Are your visuals in alignment with your feelings?

This is such a crucial question to ask yourself. If what you are feeling is not aligned with your visualization, manifesting your desires will be difficult.

For example, you cannot be asking for health and vitality in your body while your underlying belief is one of sickness. You can't be asking for abundance when the words out of your mouth are full of negativity and lack.

Remember, *faith it until you make it*. If you are asking for health, believe that you are already well. Visualize what well-being looks and feels like to you. Picture your body, your organs, and your cells operating at an optimal level; picture yourself thriving. This goes for anything you are asking the Universe for.

At times, you will become aware of energies that are blocking your desired outcome, like *un*forgiveness, jealousy, resentment, and hate. Please, please do what you need to release this type of energy from your soul, mind, and body.

This is where my daily practice and my nightly routine come into play. Before I go to sleep, I take a moment to ask and offer forgiveness for any negative behavior and thoughts I may have had about others or myself during the day. Then I go into gratitude and appreciation, and I focus on the *why* behind my gratitude and appreciation. The *why* anchors my thankfulness.

It is a great feeling to end the day with. This nightly process doesn't take a lot of time, but it gives me a moment to reset and align to my desires and visualization. My *why* for doing this is quite simple: I want what I want because I know I will feel good having it. That, however, doesn't mean I am waiting to feel good when my desire finally manifests. No!

I am feeling good *now,* feeling abundant *now,* feeling love, and being love *now,* feeling happy and thrilled *now.* Feel abundant and happy *now,* while you are looking for evidence along the way and taking the necessary inspired steps.

Aligning to your visual requires being present with your thoughts and feelings as often as you can. You will mess up sometimes. Believe me; I mess up sometimes. We all do. Learn how to reset in the way I've talked about here; establish your own nightly routine. For God's sake, and for the love of self, be gentle and loving with yourself when you make mistakes.

# CHAPTER FOUR

---

# Creating Your Life on Paper

## THE POWER OF JOURNALING

Our stories matter. They matter to us and they matter to others. Writing your story in notes or journals—or in a book like this one—can have a powerful impact. The act of writing or journaling as a tool to create can literally transform your life beyond your wildest dreams.

In writing my story, I have gained many insights into who I am and what I do, and now, it is my hope that what I have written will help you on your journey. The act of writing or journaling as a tool to create can literally transform your life beyond your wildest dreams.

### Taking Your Story Out of Your Head

Writing can be challenging. Taking my story out of my head and onto paper has certainly been a real challenge for me. Taking bits and pieces of my life to put in a book for others to read is hard. I've had to keep telling myself that what I share is important, and that the right person — you — is waiting on me. Phew — that is really good to know!

I have spent so much time in my head. I know I have talked myself out of great opportunities. There is a cheeky little voice of distraction in me that will easily give me a bag of crap. It lies to me. It is as if that voice does not want me to reach the Promised Land that I have created for myself. What a nuisance!

That voice of distraction is one reason I have become a believer in taking my story out of my head and putting it on paper. For millennials and Gen-Xers, creating a voice note on your phone or tablet may work well. I love the good old pen and paper.

Writing helps me more easily enter a world of possibility. Taking my story out of my head allows me to de-clutter my brain and gain some wisdom and clarity. It enables me to have some relief from feeling stressed, burdened, and overwhelmed by all the traffic of thoughts that might otherwise get congested into a state of worry. Writing has allowed me to freely explore my wildest dreams.

## How to Create Through Journaling

Start your writing process in a relaxed and easy way. No need to stress about it. The more relaxed and open you are, the more effective your journaling will be.

I have learned that it's best to write in such a way that makes me feel relieved and hopeful. Whenever necessary, I forgive the negative, then I self-soothe. Then, and only then, do I write my feelings around my desires, focusing on the positive. This works for me.

An alternate way is to write down everything that comes to mind in no particular order. Just get it out of your head. Once you see the words, you may find that something magical happens that inspires your writing to become more serious and more purposeful. As you write, you should notice that your mind becomes more at ease and your thoughts and emotions become clearer. During this time is when light bulbs — those ah-ha moments — often show themselves.

I have taught myself to write only what I want because that is where I want my creative energies to go. The practice brings me closer to the core feeling of joy and happiness I want to achieve; therefore, what I write becomes real.

If, instead, I were to focus on the negatives or on what I don't want — which we are so good at doing — I would get more of those same negative things.

It does help to know right off the bat what you *don't* want so you can then focus and create what you *do* want. Writing helps me figure this out. It assists me by testing my dreams and my desires. When I see what I have written on paper, I get to check in with my inner guidance to see if my words feel believable and resonate with my *why*.

If it feels believable, I usually write more details until the excitement of the desire feels as believable as if I already have it. That is my intention. That is also the fun part for me.

What do I do if what I've written isn't believable?

I abandon the thought. The reason I do this is because the vibration I get from not believing what I have written may send me into a negative thought pattern; it may make me feel unworthy of the desire. Other negative thoughts may come up based on that feeling of unworthiness.

**Let Yourself Dream**

Once you rid your mind of the weeds of life that can cripple everything — worry, fear, overwhelm, fretfulness — then you can allow myself to explore your wildest dreams. You will see the amazing possibilities that life has to offer, more than you could ever imagine.

When you are ready, you will find, as I have, that opportunities abound.

For me, I have this moment on paper when my imagination is given a green light: *Go!* I see this plain white canvas on which I get to create my dream exactly the way that I want to feel it. And in writing my dream on paper, I get to experience the sweetness and joy of it before it is even realized.

At that point, I simply allow myself to enjoy the moment. When I do this, I notice ideas popping up that lead to action steps I can take toward my dreams. These are the inspired action steps I referred to earlier.

Some of those action steps can seem small, but I know it's for me to be obedient. The importance of taking these steps, though they may seem minuscule or dumb in your mind, is showing the Universe that you are obedient, you are a believer, and you are ready. No dumb or small ideas here!

The Universe is conspiring to help you bring your desire into reality. So be obedient. Sometimes it's easier said than done, I know that for sure. But take the action step. Keep in mind that *faith without works is dead*.

Always remember and affirm that your dreams matter. Once we put those beautiful big dreams on paper, we give them life in a different way, and we never know where these dreams will take us.

## HOW TO CREATE THE LIFE YOU WANT

How do you create the life you want in a relaxed and easy way? We'll talk more about that here.

### Know What You Want

First, get clear on what you want. Only then will the Universe know what you want.

Imagine if I asked you what you want, and you shrugged your shoulders and said, "I don't know."

If I wanted to give you a gift, I would not know what to give you. Let the Universe know what you want.

The truth is that I think you do know what you want, but you may have a belief that says *I probably can't get it*. You may have told yourself you are not worthy or deserving. You may be thinking you can't make a living doing this thing you want to do.

Guess what?

Lies, lies, and more lies.

What is the one thing you would love to be doing?

Be honest and take money out of the equation. At Christmas, kids usually give their parents a list of what they want and they are usually quite clear and descriptive. Some may even include a picture. They know what they want down to the very last detail. They usually feel energized and excited about it, and when they think on it, they feel very happy. When writing their wish lists, most kids don't care about being worthy; they don't care about what others think.

That is the feeling you are after when you are trying to get clear on what you want. Find the courage to say what it is you are wishing for. Look for the energy that makes you feel full and abundant, not the one that makes you feel empty and lacking. You deserve what you want and you deserve to feel good about it.

## The *Why*

Next, get clear on why you want what you want. That *why* is going to anchor your commitment to your desires.

The *why* for me is an emotion, a feeling coming from my heart and soul. The *why* should feel expansive and full of possibility; it should be thrilling. If the *why* pulls you down and makes you feel low or unworthy, you will not — I repeat, you will not — be able to get clear or commit. You will not have enough courage and belief to manifest what you truly desire.

Your *why* will also get you through moments when you want to give up. In that moment, a quick pause to go back to your *why* will have you rethink that desire to quit and keep you moving forward.

Now the *why*, as I see it, is always associated with a feeling that comes from within your heart and soul. This feeling is an emotion that connects you to what you want.

For example, suppose I want to release excess weight from my body. My *why* is that I deserve to feel good about myself, to feel vibrant and full of energy, to feel my best. I deserve to feel good in my clothes. I deserve to feel happy and healthy. I deserve to feel well. That is my *why*. I can actually feel my *why* because it is connected to my heart and soul.

When you know what you want, figure out your *why* before you move forward, and be sure it is connected to your heart and soul.

## The *How*

So many times, the *how* is what stops us dead in our tracks before we even make an attempt. We get so caught up in trying to figure out the *how* that we just revert or run away. We succumb to the notion that what we want will never happen for us—before we even try. We say *it's too hard, we're too old, we're too young*, or *there's not enough money*. The *how* has been given the power to paralyze us from moving toward what we truly desire.

*How* is a logical question and one we've been trained to ask. However, the truth is how stuff happens is really none of our business. I have come to believe that we need God, the Universe—or whatever we call that invisible resource or inner guide in our lives—to help us in co-creating our big audacious dreams.

God's dream for me is so much bigger than I can dream.

What I know for sure is that God is able to do "exceedingly abundantly above all that we can ask or think, according to the power that works in us." (Ephesians 3:20, KJV).

Do you believe this?

If you don't, then you might as well not dream because the *how* is inevitably going to stifle the dream. In addition, when you are focused on the *how*, the heavy lifting will be all yours, along with a series of daunting action steps that truly do not support who you are.

It doesn't have to be that way. The Universe knows exactly how to get you to your destination, your desire. These journeys won't rely exclusively on your strength; you won't have to do all the heavy lifting. You will find that people and opportunities will turn up to support you and help you get to your destination.

Look back to the example I gave about my trip to Europe. That trip would not have happened without the support of the Divine. If I had gotten caught up with the *how*, I would have had to generate so much business to make enough money, and that would have stressed me out like crazy. My experience would not have been what I wanted; in fact, the trip probably would not have happened at all.

Instead of focusing on the *how*, all I did was keep moving as I felt inspired. I did all I could do on my end and left the heavy lifting to the Universe. And I wasn't disappointed at all. I didn't have to compete or push anyone out of the way to get what I wanted. All I did was keep my desire alive, have fun, and serve my clients and myself well.

## THE VALUE OF APPRECIATION AND GRATITUDE

Is there a difference between appreciation and gratitude?

*Gratitude* is defined in the Oxford dictionary as "the quality of being thankful; readiness to show appreciation for and to return kindness."

*Appreciation* is defined in the Oxford dictionary as "the recognition and enjoyment of the good qualities of someone or something," while The Miriam Webster dictionary defines it as "the act of recognizing and understanding that something is valuable, important."

With all the research I have done, what actually resonates with me is this relationship between appreciation and gratitude. Gratitude demonstrates a readiness to show appreciation. Appreciation deepens gratitude. As Deborah Price wrote, "Gratitude is a base from which appreciation grows and flourishes if we pay attention."[7]

We know that people can say thank you and be grateful even when they don't necessarily appreciate you or your gifts. Appreciating something or someone involves a shift for me, a deepening of my thankfulness.

In the same article quoted above, Ms. Price went on to state, "The subtle shift from gratitude to appreciation involves being more present, more thoughtfully aware and active in reflecting on the reasons we feel grateful about something or someone."[8]

---

7 Price, Deborah. "Gratitude and Appreciation: What's the Difference?" Beliefnet.com, 2009. beliefnet.com/columnists/yourdailyspiritualstimulus/2009/04/gratitude-and-appreciation-whats-the-difference.html
8 Price, 2009.

Being in gratitude takes practice, and so does appreciation. Both of them require that we increase our awareness and consciousness. Below is a helpful exercise that I do myself, and also teach to my clients.

To foster gratitude and appreciation:

- Focus on an object, an experience, or a person and visualize.

- Ask yourself why you feel grateful for this.

- Use the *why* to anchor the gratitude in the moment.

- Allow yourself to appreciate the characteristics that you are grateful for.

For example, I can be grateful for having clothes to wear. I can think of many reasons. The *why* anchors the gratitude in the moment and brings me into a state of awareness, more heart-centered than in the conscious mind. I can take it a step further by appreciating the beauty and style of the clothes, how well they fit my body, the ease of wearing them, and how confident I feel. Appreciation allows me to move beyond my mind, my consciousness; it allows me to recognize the value the clothes bring to my life.

## The Small Things Matter

Often, it is the little things in life that ma\
*Appreciate what we have. Be grateful.* I have
words many times, and they are great a      .ve
can all appreciate the little signs; we can see them as
breadcrumbs along the way to our desires. It is the
little signs along the way that keep me going; they give
me a God-wink that tells me I am on the right path.

When I have a dream and I am visualizing, I get
excited when I come across evidence that reminds me
of my desire. For example, perhaps I have intended
a week of feeling abundant. That abundance could
mean many things: unexpected money, new business,
new relationships, and so on. When I say *I am feeling
abundant,* I commit to being present while I look for
evidence, signals, or clues that tell me I am getting
closer to realizing the abundance.

I may notice coins on the street and I will pick them
up and give thanks. I may meet new people and I
will appreciate the experience and the person because
it is practice for what is to come: the main event I
am always looking forward to. I love nature, trees
especially, and when I see fluffy, beautiful, big trees,
the leaves remind of the Universe's expansiveness and
abundance. I cannot count those leaves, so I imagine
that expansiveness and abundance is mine.

ᴧcknowledging and appreciating those small nuggets lets the Universe know that I want more and I'm ready for more. Small experiences acknowledged in the hands of a big God can and will make a big difference.

## Be Aware of How You're Feeling Moment to Moment

This journey of life is just that: a journey to a destination. It's a journey to a destination that we hope, believe, and trust will bring us everlasting joy. But it is on the road we travel where the happiness, joy, and excitement are supposed to be experienced.

We have a choice to be present with how we are feeling in every moment — or not to be present. Hey, I get that life happens, but we *always* have that choice to be present. It is this presence, this state of being, that can propel us quickly to the pot of gold at the end of the rainbow. Or we can stay stuck in the unhappiness we don't seem to want to let go of. Being aware, moment by moment, is key to all aspects of our lives.

For example, when you are experiencing strong feelings, do you have the ability to stay present and aware, and to keep from lashing out?

Yes, you do. You can choose your response, and that is key to being an outstanding leader in business and in the leadership of your life. As Janet Britcher wrote, "With some vigilance, impulsive reactions and comments of the *blurt and hurt* variety can be managed without losing the benefits of awareness."[9]

Truth is, I am really working on this area of my being. I am not at all saying you should sweep feelings under the rug. I am saying that, to be effective in any given moment with your emotions is to be aware of them. You can acknowledge them, reflect on their sources and meaning, and choose your response. I like to call this response *pause*.

*Pause* long enough to acknowledge your feelings. Move from old response patterns that never bear good fruit.

Seek a better perspective of the situation. Emotional reactions can be a source of information and wisdom if we are open. Look at the situation as is, making sure you are not discrediting or disallowing your feelings. Then look at the situation from a distance to see the whole, and possibly a differing, perspective before you determine the response to the situation. The *pause* really makes a world of difference in diffusing strong feelings you may have in that moment.

---

9 Britcher, Janet. "Why Being Aware of Your Feelings Is Key to Outstanding Leadership." Forbes.com, Nov. 15, 2018. forbes.com/sites/forbescoachescouncil/2018/11/15/why-being-aware-of-your-feelings-is-key-to-outstanding-leadership

# CHAPTER FIVE

---

# Is Your Perspective Serving You Well?

## SHIFTING NEGATIVE EXPERIENCES INTO A BETTER FEELING

The word *perspective* "has a Latin root, meaning 'look through' or 'perceive,' and all the meanings of perspective have something to do with looking." (Vocabulary.com)

For me, *perspective* is how I see something in any given moment, and, on a deeper level, how I feel about what I am looking at. When your perspective is negative, it impacts everything in your life, so finding a new perspective can be miraculous. You could go from *everything is happening to me* to *everything is happening for me,* from *sickness* to *wellness,* from *lack* to *abundance.*

How can you change perspective?

How can you see and feel things differently and be in gratitude all at the same time? Is this really doable?

Yes. Take your time with the process. Stop right now, and take three deep breaths slowly: inhale slowly and exhale slowly. Honor what is, and what is around us in the moment.

## Asking Questions Can Bring New Perspectives

Questions are a natural part of communication. We can use them to get information from each other, but they can also help us get answers from ourselves and can help us shift perspective.

The key is — how good is the question you are asking? Are you asking the right questions?

Asking good questions helps us take ownership of what we want, what we want to know, and what we want to experience. My intent for this section of this book is for you, my beloved, to start to question or communicate with yourself, your inner being, first.

No matter what the situation is, this begins with asking God, the Holy Spirit, the Divine — or whatever you call your inner guide — these two questions:

1. How can I see this differently?
2. How do I want to feel right now?

These two questions come back to the simple need to love on yourself in that very moment. You want to feel better. If you feel distressed, scared, anxious, or whatever that not-so-good feeling is, you can change that feeling, as well as your reaction to it.

*How can I see this differently?* By asking this first question, we are seeking a new improved perspective that allows peace to come into our hearts.

*How do I want to feel right now?* We've talked about the importance of being aware of your feelings at any given moment. Being aware requires that you are present and that you acknowledge your feelings, your energy, and your vibes. Although *How do I want to feel right now?* may seem like a simple question, it isn't always that straightforward or easy to answer when you are faced with a challenging situation, a hardship, a sadness, or a tragedy. I know this to be true.

When I was faced with having to take care of both of my parents, who are at different ages and stages of declining health, I had a difficult time answering that question. I'm their only child here in Jamaica; my only other sibling resides in the United States. Initially, I felt overwhelmed.

I asked: *How can I find a different perspective of this situation that makes me feel better, despite how it looks to the naked eye?*

Trust me; this has been very hard. It took me a better part of a year to realize that feeling stressed, upset, angry, distraught, sad, and depressed at this situation I found myself in wasn't serving me well at all.

You may ask how I knew it wasn't serving me well. The answer is I felt like shit — physically, mentally, and emotionally. I wanted to give up on myself and on them; I wanted to quit. And it started to manifest in my body, resulting in a decline in my own health and vitality. The weight of this burden — and yes, that is how I felt, no judgment here please — literally manifested itself inside and outside of my body. Weight gain was one of the symptoms, an ultra-representation of the heaviness I felt inside.

I found myself asking the question: *Why me?*

In that moment, it felt like my life, as I knew it, was over, but that wasn't the case. On the contrary, I got to press the reset button and rewrite the rest of my story.

## Acknowledge Your Fears

From the question: *How do I want to feel right now?* comes the thought, hopefully, of wanting to feel better. Inherently we want to have an improved feeling, even if that improved feeling is ever so slightly better than the current feeling of despair, sadness, hurt, or anger.

The truth we need to acknowledge is that these feelings are all coming from one source: fear. Fear of the unknown. Fear of failure. Fear of loss. Fear of not being good enough. Fear of unworthiness. Fear of not deserving the best. Fear of being alone. This *fear of* list can go on forever.

The fears that went along with being caregiver to both my parents were:

- Not good enough to do this
- Not having enough resources to take care of them
- Not being able to live and enjoy my life anymore
- Having to live with them
- Failing at this thing called *life*

Remember that *failure at life* was a fear I had when I left high school without a diploma. The more dominant that fear was, the more I began to fear the future, the unknown, and a scarcity of resources—specifically money. It was as if the abundance mindset that I had spent so much time developing went through the door. I went into such a place of feeling that there wouldn't be enough. My faith felt like it sprouted wings and flew away, and I found myself completely out of whack.

My energies were all over the place, and I simply didn't feel good. I experienced weight gain and sleepless nights and felt miserable most of the time. I was snapping at other people and getting pissed off easily. In the moment, those feelings seemed easy and logical; besides, I had practiced them for so long.

As humans, we somehow have been socialized to stay in these negative feelings for long periods. We tend to talk about them over and over. You might even feel a strange sense of satisfaction and normalcy in feeling lousy. But we never have to settle for lousy. We can choose to reach out for a better feeling.

## Reach for a Better Feeling

Ask the question: *How do I want to feel right now?*

From the *ask,* reach for that better feeling via a change in the space if you can. Take in a deep purposeful breath and, counting to ten or to a hundred, allow a new thought or perspective to form so you can simply feel a little better. In some cases, this will happen quickly; in other instances, it will take some time. Please be gentle and loving with yourself. Seek out gratitude and appreciation.

When it seems challenging to get a new perspective on a situation or to be grateful, I allow myself to reach for a thought or a picture of a time when I experienced a good or better feeling. It may be as simple as remembering a time when I laughed really hard.

If I can see trees or other forms of nature, I will look at them and will soon feel the energy of abundance or resilience slowly replacing negative energies. The trees I see stand tall even in the face of hardships. The leaves for me represent abundance, and when the leaves move, I believe they are smiling and dancing with me. That is my go-to.

I can be like the trees and bloom where I am planted. It's a choice. You, too, can bloom where you are planted.

I am planted in that power within me; it is the soil I get to shine from. I always have the choice to reset and renew, so I can go into the space of being grateful and appreciate the moment for what it is. At the end of the day, I am reaching for peace, knowing I did the best I could.

What are you reaching for?

## Affirming the Truth of Who We Are

Reaching for a better feeling is just the beginning. Now you get to decide and affirm your belief around the improved feeling, your desire, and what you deserve. In essence, you now need to water the better feeling with affirmations, self-love, and people who will support your new norm—the new improved feeling that you desire and deserve.

It is in this moment of affirming your truth—the authentic truth that rings true for you, the truth you can believe about yourself without a doubt—that you will begin to allow your life to shine.

*You don't have to worry about what their vibration is if your vibration is one of connection. Because if your vibration is one of connection you are going to dominate the vibration.*[10]

~ Abraham Hicks

In this process, there is no fighting with the situation or with unwanted feelings. You are not trying to flee from it or run away from it; you are reaching for a better feeling. Be honest with yourself here. The honesty will lead to sustainable positive change in an easy and relaxed way.

Also, please be gentle with yourself. Don't bully yourself by repeating scolding words like these: *You need to be positive! You need to get positive!*

Instead, ask that simple question: *How do I want to feel right now?*

The idea here is to remind you of your power. That power within you allows your light to shine so brightly.

10 Hicks, Abraham. Facebook.com, Jan. 14, 2013. facebook.com/
Abraham.Hicks/posts/you-dont-have-to-worry-about-what-
their-vibration-is-if-your-vibration-is-one-of/447257528734241

Be vulnerable with your truth. Surrender in the moment so that power, that light, can come through you to show you the way to the improved feeling.

## PERSONAL ACCOUNTABILITY: OWNING YOUR ACTIONS

Taking ownership of your own actions and words, even when it means admitting you made a mistake, even if you feel like a failure, is essential to personal growth. This is such a challenge for many of us, myself included. We must all strive for accountability.

> *Good men are bound by conscience and*
> *liberated by accountability.*[11]
>
> ~ Wes Fesler

For simplicity, accountability means being of your word, seeing through what you said you would do. My father used to say, "A man's word is his bond." In his mind, there was an implicit trust associated with one's words. Fast-forward to current times and it seems we don't have that same unshakeable trust in the words of others, or of ourselves. Let's return to those ideals.

Shelby Martin said, "Personal accountability requires mindfulness, acceptance, honesty, and courage," and

11 inspiringquotes.us/author/2494-wes-fesler/about-conscience

I believe this to be true.[12] Acceptance and ownership of what is happening often takes courage, and being aware and present is necessary to allow a solution to come in. Yes, accountability and ownership require consciousness, openness, and vulnerability.

## Whom Am I Blaming?

*"If you could kick the person in the pants responsible for most of your trouble, you wouldn't sit for a month."*
~ attributed to Theodore Roosevelt

For many of us, a barrier to accountability is *blame*. We often start blaming others for circumstances in hope that this strategy will help things get better. Unfortunately, when we blame others, we give up the power to change and improve.

Failure and mistakes are simply a part of life. Let's just breathe that in and bring acceptance.

## Accountability, Responsibility, and Ownership

*Give someone responsibility and they will do their best. Make them accountable and they will do even better.[13]*
~ Simon Sinek

---

12 Martin, Shelby. "Personal Accountability." *Libero Magazine.* Oct. 30, 2014. liberomagazine.com/eatingdisorders/personal-accountability
13 Twitter, @simonsinek accessed 02/12/09 at 3:25pm.

Responsibility and ownership are a part of being accountable.

Simply put, we accept responsibility for our actions. We are accountable for our results. We take ownership of our mistakes.

That's it, in a nutshell.

## Own Up When You Mess Up: Don't Give Away Your Power

Being accountable can be one of the biggest keys to happiness.

I am not saying this because it sounds good or because it is easy. I am saying this because owning my actions when I mess up gives me a much better feeling than giving away my power and my control to someone else because I could not accept and own my mistake.

Let's go back to my story about not getting a diploma from high school. In retrospect, as I think back to that time, it was right for me to own and accept that I flopped the religious studies exam. It doesn't matter whether it was because I didn't apply myself to that subject or I did not understand it. I failed, and the consequence was a school-leaving certificate. At that time, it meant that I was not good enough; I was a failure. I felt ashamed and unsupported.

At some point, I must have taken ownership of my failure because the right people turned up to help me get to the next level—my acceptance to Rutgers University. Own your weaknesses and no one will have control of you. Own your insecurities and your mistakes in life, and you can forgive yourself and move forward. The more you practice this, the easier it will get. You will find that life will support you. Those blunders may turn out to be the forces that bring out your greatest strengths.

## Accept the Truth and Choose Your Response

It is okay to feel shame, disgrace, and hopelessness. We all have those feelings sometimes. During the low times I've shared with you, I called myself all sorts of names.

It is okay to feel disappointed, but to destroy yourself is not the answer. I wouldn't recommend you build a home in disappointment. It doesn't serve anyone, least of all yourself. *You have to be your biggest fan.*

When you make a mistake, first accept what is. Then, choose a better response and move forward. Being able to accept what is allows a different response that is usually more favorable for a better outcome.

Being your biggest fan doesn't mean ignoring your mistakes. It means saying to yourself: *I am worth it and*

*I deserve this,* even when you have made a mistake. You have to believe that you are worthy even if you mess up. Yes, it may hurt in the moment. You may feel disappointed and you may beat on yourself a bit, but only for a moment. Switch it up as fast as you can to a more-improved place.

Now let's be clear. I have had moments when I couldn't shake the feeling of disappointment or accept what is. When this happens, what I do is honor my feelings and then press a reset button before going to bed with the intention that tomorrow will be a good day. If I don't do this, disappointment snowballs into a big mess and negative feelings take over. That simply sucks. Just saying!

Remember, your energy is your responsibility. You deserve to feel good despite the messes that you must own.

## HOW FULL IS YOUR GLASS?

Is your glass half full? Is it half empty?

The question is used to remind us how we're looking at life, and my answer is this: No matter how I look at my glass, I certainly have more than enough for now.

It depends on how you want to see it; your perspective represents your view of the world.

## Giving From the Overflow

Either viewpoint can be good, depending on your perspective.

I like to think of this in terms of *giving* and *receiving*.

If I have given of myself emotionally, physically, and materialistically, I have empty space left, which allows me to be open to receive. By *open to receive*, I mean there is a space available to allow self-care and self-love. It means taking time to replenish.

The truth is we all should be giving from the overflow. I have more than enough for my needs; indeed, "my cup overflows." (Psalm 23:5, NIV)

I don't want anyone reading this who has a different perspective on the *glass-half-empty-or-full* question to feel wronged in any way; it is your view. However, if I can be so bold, if I can help you to have a better perspective on whatever your glass represents, that is my intention. Be open to seeing something better. It is difficult and challenging to get through life successfully with a *glass-half-empty* mindset.

It all comes back, as you probably noticed, to the aspects of your life where we can find light and hope. Wherever we find light and hope, we find more in the blessings of giving thanks. Get into gratitude and see how that little hope or light grows in that moment.

## Mindfulness: Keeping an Eye on Your Glass

When was the last time you got out of your bed and decided you were going to have a good day, no matter what?

The *no matter what* part is a promise to stay present in each moment of the day, but then — guess what? Some curveball hits you out of nowhere and it knocks the *having a good day* right out of you. At that point, frustration, impatience, or rage will run right in.

Natural emotions one would have, right?

Yes, and it is easy to respond to the curveball in a way you never intended. You truly have two choices in this moment. You can change to a more pleasant feeling, or you can remain in an unpleasant state and have it snowball into a much worse feeling.

Have you ever responded to something unpleasant by allowing yourself to sink into a crappy, negative mood and then see your day become a day from hell?

For me, that is a resounding yes. And the truth is, when it's so bad, the only thing I can do is forget the day and sleep it off with the hope and intention of having a better day tomorrow. *Easier said than done* may be what you are thinking, and that's okay. But I can share with you what I do in these easy steps.

First, you have to want to feel better. That is key, and that is your choice to have.

So, if that is your intention, before you go to bed:

1.  Acknowledge the day for what it was. Bless it, thank it, and wish it well.

2.  Forgive yourself and others; be gentle with yourself in this moment.

3.  Intend a better day tomorrow.

4.  Find one-to-three things you can be grateful for, like the comfort of your bed or simply having a bed, a good night's sleep, food to eat, being able to take a bath, running water, electricity.

5.  Go to sleep.

These five steps give you a simple reset that will help you care for yourself and keep your glass full.

In the third step, in which I advise you decide on a better tomorrow, I realize that the issue, problem, or person who is troubling you may still be there tomorrow. However, *you have the power to choose how you want to feel about it.* Look for the lessons to help you have a better day.

One of the biggest lessons I've had to learn when facing a problem or challenge is not to react quickly. Reacting quickly sends me into emotions that I often don't want or like. So, I have to — and I mean, *have to* — slow down, pause, and ask that question. By now, you should know the question I am referring to.

Yes. *How do I want to feel right now?*

You have just been purposeful in wanting to feel better, and in turn, you will have a better-feeling day tomorrow. At times, I will journal the first four steps. Writing helps me shift my perspective to the telling of a different story. Remember, all we have now is this moment.

## Keeping Your Glass Full: Paying Attention to Self

Keeping an eye on your glass takes mindfulness. That is the trick!

*Mindfulness,* per the Oxford dictionary, means:

1. The quality or state of being conscious or aware of something.

2. A mental state achieved by focusing one's awareness on the present moment, while calmly acknowledging and accepting one's feelings, thoughts, and bodily sensations, used as a therapeutic technique.

In summary, be alive in the moment, in any given moment, and be purposeful about that alignment. Most of us—a great percentage of the world—have been just existing and experiencing life as it comes our way without being mindful about how life makes us feel and how our actions are being affected by others.

It is like accepting an old situation because we assume it's not going to change whether we see the glass as half empty or half full. I beg to differ. You may not always be able to have a different perspective. I am not saying you must be present all the time, 24/7, but if you give yourself the chance, the space, and the opportunity to be present with your yucky, not-so-good feelings and be gentle with yourself in that moment to want to feel better, you can open up to allow goodness to seep into your energy.

There will be days when you aren't feeling good, when you are drained, and your mind is asking: *What's the point?*

Take a moment to inhale a very deep breath while asking yourself: *How can I feel better about this?*

You will be amazed by what is presented to you. Give it a try.

It is really worth it to take that pause, to breathe, and to ask. Please be curious, open, gentle, and accepting with respect to these new discoveries. They will assist you in keeping your glass full and help you shift your attention and your focus to something infinitely better.

# Conclusion

Reader, I want you to know that it is never too late to improve, grow, and transform. The Universe really doesn't know time the way we do. Our beliefs and our vibrations will determine whether what we desire will be slow or fast in manifesting. It is all about you. This journey is yours.

You may have to move, shift, or swerve from folks in your life who do not support your decision to improve, grow, and transform. Misery loves company, as they say. I hope you choose you. I hope you watch your life, your whole life, improve, grow, and transform in a simply easy, fun relaxed way.

During and after the reading of this book, take some time to absorb and digest the little nuggets presented, one nugget at a time. You can do this. You deserve this. You are worth it. I am here to support and honor you through this. See the next page for my contact information. You can visit my website to get information, and feel free to email me.

This book is a simple read but will have you imagining whether you can actually take this one small step toward making your life better. Please take that step.

Send me an email and share with me how this book has helped you.

I wish you joy and an abundance of blessings!

# Next Steps

Schedule a free 15-minute discovery to briefly discuss your needs and see if we are a fit for each other.

Visit my website: simplyreal.me, or email me at karla@ simplyreal.me.

# About the Author

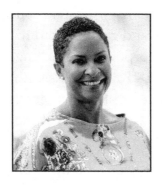

Karla Henry, BA, MSW, Certified Holistic Health Coach.

Karla graduated from the Institute for Integrative Nutrition as a Certified Holistic Health Coach, where she studied and learned innovative coaching methods, practical lifestyle coaching, and management techniques. With her knowledge and guidance, she cocreates completely personalized actions based on her clients' intentions. She will move you toward your ideal vision of a whole you, with a focus on both personal and professional lifestyle preferences.

As a coach, Karla Henry puts the power back in your hands by supporting you in improving the nutrition of your mind.

Her education has equipped her with extensive, cutting-edge knowledge of holistic nutrition for your whole life plate—health, relationships (family, friendships, romance), career/business, finances, spirituality, fun, and relationship to self. Drawing on her expertise—corporate, coaching, mental health, entrepreneurship—Karla works with clients as a guide to help them make lifestyle changes and choose health-promoting ways, via their own minds, which produce real and lasting results.

Her unique way starts with understanding what makes you do what you do, how you think, and what you believe. Her approach is to coach from a place of keeping it Simply Real. She's direct in her approach with a big dose of love.

Karla currently lives in Kingston, Jamaica. She has two degrees: a bachelor's degree in marketing from Rutgers University in New Jersey, and a master's degree in clinical social work from Barry University in Florida. Karla is also cofounder and director of a mortgage brokerage business in Jamaica called Lead Mortgage Brokers.

Made in the USA
Las Vegas, NV
07 July 2021